The Natural Path
to
Healing your Muscles

By Luna Parnell

Table of Content

Introduction

Welcome to our comprehensive guide, "The Natural Path to Healing Your Muscles." We invite you to embark on a transformative journey towards vibrant muscle health and vitality. Just as muscles are the engines that drive our bodies, they are also a reflection of our overall well-being—strong, resilient, and full of vitality.

In the pages that follow, we will delve deep into the intricate world of muscles, exploring their diverse types, essential connective tissues, and the interconnectedness of body and mind. From the powerful skeletal muscles that enable movement to the rhythmic contractions of the heart and the smooth muscles that regulate internal processes, we will unravel the mysteries of muscle function and vitality.

But our journey goes beyond mere anatomy and physiology. We will also explore the holistic principles of muscle care, embracing natural remedies, nourishment, and lifestyle practices that support optimal muscle health and performance. By harnessing the healing power of nature and embracing a holistic approach to wellness, we can unlock the innate potential within our muscles and foster strength, resilience, and vitality from within.

So, whether you're an athlete striving for peak performance, a fitness enthusiast seeking to maximize gains, or simply someone who values vibrant health and vitality, join us on this journey towards vibrant muscle health and holistic well-being. Together, let's unlock the power within and embrace a life filled with strength, resilience, and radiant vitality.

Welcome to "The Natural Path to Healing Your Muscles." Let the journey begin.

The Muscular System

The muscular system is a complex network of tissues that allows the body to move, maintain posture, and circulate blood and other substances. It consists of three main types of muscles: skeletal, cardiac, and smooth muscles. Each type of muscle has distinct characteristics and functions.

Types of Muscles

Skeletal Muscles:

- Structure: Long, cylindrical fibers with multiple nuclei per cell. They have a striated (striped) appearance due to the organized arrangement of actin and myosin filaments.
- Function: Voluntary movement of the body, posture maintenance, heat production.
- Control: Voluntary (somatic nervous system).
- Location: Attached to bones by tendons.
- Examples: Biceps brachii, quadriceps, hamstrings.

Cardiac Muscle:

- Structure: Short, branched fibers with a single central nucleus per cell. Striated appearance similar to skeletal muscle, with intercalated discs that connect adjacent cells.
- Function: Pumps blood throughout the body.
- Control: Involuntary (autonomic nervous system).
- Location: Walls of the heart (myocardium).

Smooth Muscles:

- Structure: Spindle-shaped fibers with a single central nucleus per cell. Non-striated appearance due to the random arrangement of actin and myosin filaments.
- Function: Moves substances through internal organs, regulates blood vessel diameter.
- Control: Involuntary (autonomic nervous system).
- Location: Walls of internal organs and blood vessels.

- Examples: Muscles in the digestive tract, blood vessels, bladder.

Muscle Fiber Types in Skeletal Muscles

- Type I (Slow-Twitch Fibers):
    - Characteristics: High endurance, fatigue-resistant, more mitochondria, high myoglobin content (red fibers).
    - Function: Sustained, low-intensity activities (e.g., long-distance running).
- Type IIa (Fast-Twitch Oxidative Fibers):
    - Characteristics: Intermediate endurance, some fatigue resistance, moderate mitochondria and myoglobin content.
    - Function: Medium-duration activities (e.g., middle-distance running).
- Type IIb (Fast-Twitch Glycolytic Fibers):
    - Characteristics: Low endurance, quick to fatigue, fewer mitochondria, low myoglobin content (white fibers).

- Function: Short, high-intensity
  activities (e.g., sprinting,
  weightlifting).

Structure of Skeletal Muscle

- Muscle Fiber (Cell):
    - Myofibrils: Rod-like units within
      muscle fibers containing
      sarcomeres.
    - Sarcomeres: The basic contractile
      units of muscle fibers, composed
      of actin (thin filaments) and
      myosin (thick filaments).
    - Sarcolemma: Plasma membrane
      of a muscle fiber.
    - Sarcoplasm: Cytoplasm of a
      muscle fiber.
    - Sarcoplasmic Reticulum:
      Specialized endoplasmic
      reticulum that stores calcium
      ions.
- Connective Tissue Layers:
    - Endomysium: Surrounds
      individual muscle fibers.
    - Perimysium: Surrounds bundles
      of muscle fibers (fascicles).

- Epimysium: Surrounds the entire muscle.

Muscle Contraction Mechanism

- Neuromuscular Junction: The synapse between a motor neuron and a muscle fiber.
- Action Potential: Electrical signal transmitted by the motor neuron.
- Release of Acetylcholine: Neurotransmitter released at the neuromuscular junction.
- Muscle Fiber Excitation: Depolarization of the sarcolemma.
- Calcium Release: From the sarcoplasmic reticulum into the sarcoplasm.
- Cross-Bridge Formation: Myosin heads bind to actin filaments.
- Power Stroke: Myosin heads pivot, pulling actin filaments toward the center of the sarcomere.
- ATP Binding: Causes myosin heads to detach from actin and reset.

Muscle Functions

- Movement: Skeletal muscles contract to produce movement of bones and body parts.
- Posture: Muscles work continuously to maintain body posture.
- Heat Production: Muscle activity generates heat, contributing to body temperature regulation.
- Circulation: Cardiac muscle contractions pump blood; smooth muscles in blood vessels regulate blood flow.
- Respiration: Diaphragm and intercostal muscles enable breathing.

Integration with Other Systems

- Nervous System: Controls muscle contraction through motor neurons and neuromuscular junctions.
- Skeletal System: Provides attachment points and levers for muscle action.
- Cardiovascular System: Supplies oxygen and nutrients to muscles, removes metabolic waste.
- Respiratory System: Delivers oxygen to muscles, removes carbon dioxide.
- Endocrine System: Hormones regulate muscle growth, metabolism, and repair.

The muscular system is a highly specialized network essential for voluntary and involuntary movements, posture, and vital functions. Understanding its components, including the different types of muscles and their specific roles, provides a foundation for appreciating the complexity and efficiency of human movement and bodily function.

Skeletal Muscles

Skeletal muscles are one of the three major muscle types in the human body, the others being cardiac and smooth muscles. They are crucial for voluntary movements, posture maintenance, and overall bodily functions. Here, we'll explore the structure, function, types, and mechanisms of skeletal muscles in detail.

Structure of Skeletal Muscles

Muscle Fiber (Cell):

- Myofibrils: Each muscle fiber contains numerous myofibrils, which are rod-like structures composed of repeating units called sarcomeres.
- Sarcomeres: The basic contractile units of muscle fibers, made up of actin (thin filaments) and myosin (thick filaments). The arrangement of these filaments gives skeletal muscles their striated appearance.
- Sarcolemma: The plasma membrane of a muscle fiber that encloses the sarcoplasm.

- Sarcoplasm: The cytoplasm of a muscle fiber, containing organelles, myofibrils, glycogen, and myoglobin.
- Sarcoplasmic Reticulum (SR): A specialized type of smooth endoplasmic reticulum that stores and releases calcium ions, which are essential for muscle contraction.
- T-tubules (Transverse Tubules): Invaginations of the sarcolemma that help transmit action potentials deep into the muscle fiber, ensuring coordinated contractions.

Connective Tissue Layers:

- Endomysium: A delicate layer of connective tissue that surrounds each individual muscle fiber.
- Perimysium: A thicker layer of connective tissue that surrounds bundles of muscle fibers, known as fascicles.
- Epimysium: The outermost layer of dense connective tissue that surrounds the entire muscle, providing protection and structural support.
- Tendons: Connective tissues that attach muscles to bones, transmitting the force

generated by muscle contractions to produce movement.

Function of Skeletal Muscles

1. Movement: Skeletal muscles contract to pull on bones, generating movement at joints. This includes actions such as walking, running, lifting, and manipulating objects.
2. Posture: Continuous, low-level contractions of skeletal muscles maintain body posture and stability.
3. Heat Production: Muscle contractions generate heat as a byproduct, helping to maintain body temperature.
4. Protection: Skeletal muscles provide padding and support for internal organs.
5. Metabolic Functions: Muscles store glycogen and can perform gluconeogenesis, contributing to overall energy metabolism.

Types of Skeletal Muscle Fibers

1. Type I (Slow-Twitch Fibers):
   - Characteristics: High endurance, fatigue-resistant, contain more mitochondria, high myoglobin content (red fibers).
   - Function: Suitable for sustained, low-intensity activities such as long-distance running and maintaining posture.
   - Energy Source: Aerobic respiration.
2. Type IIa (Fast-Twitch Oxidative Fibers):
   - Characteristics: Intermediate endurance, moderately fatigue-resistant, moderate mitochondria and myoglobin content.
   - Function: Suitable for medium-duration activities such as middle-distance running and swimming.
   - Energy Source: Combination of aerobic and anaerobic respiration.
3. Type IIb (Fast-Twitch Glycolytic Fibers):
   - Characteristics: Low endurance, quickly fatigued, fewer

mitochondria, low myoglobin
content (white fibers).

- Function: Suitable for short,
  high-intensity activities such as
  sprinting and weightlifting.
- Energy Source: Anaerobic
  respiration.

Mechanism of Muscle Contraction

1. Neuromuscular Junction: The site
   where a motor neuron communicates
   with a muscle fiber.
2. Action Potential: An electrical signal
   from the motor neuron triggers the
   release of acetylcholine (ACh) into the
   synaptic cleft.
3. ACh Binding: ACh binds to receptors on
   the muscle fiber's sarcolemma, causing
   depolarization and generating an action
   potential in the muscle fiber.
4. T-tubules and SR Interaction: The
   action potential travels along the
   sarcolemma and down T-tubules,
   triggering the release of calcium ions
   from the SR.
5. Calcium Binding: Calcium ions bind to
   troponin, causing a conformational

change that moves tropomyosin away from actin's myosin-binding sites.

6. Cross-Bridge Cycling: Myosin heads bind to actin, forming cross-bridges. Using ATP, myosin heads pivot, pulling actin filaments toward the center of the sarcomere (power stroke).

7. ATP Role: ATP binds to myosin, causing it to detach from actin and reset for another cycle.

8. Muscle Relaxation: When neural stimulation ceases, calcium ions are pumped back into the SR, and tropomyosin covers actin's binding sites, stopping the contraction.

Herbs, Minerals, and Vitamins for Skeletal Muscle Health

Maintaining healthy skeletal muscles requires a combination of proper nutrition, adequate exercise, and sometimes supplemental support through herbs, minerals, and vitamins. Below is a detailed list of key nutrients and herbs that contribute to the formation, maintenance, and healing of skeletal muscles, along with their specific benefits and sources.

Vitamins

1. Vitamin D
    - Function: Essential for muscle function and strength. Enhances calcium absorption, which is crucial for muscle contraction.
    - Sources: Sunlight, fatty fish (salmon, mackerel), fortified dairy products, and supplements.
2. Vitamin C
    - Function: Important for collagen synthesis, which supports muscle structure and repair. Acts as an antioxidant, protecting muscles from damage.
    - Sources: Citrus fruits, strawberries, bell peppers, broccoli, and supplements.
3. Vitamin E
    - Function: Antioxidant that helps prevent oxidative stress and muscle damage during exercise.
    - Sources: Nuts, seeds, spinach, and vegetable oils.

4. B Vitamins (B6, B12, Folate)
    - Function: Support energy production and red blood cell formation, which is essential for oxygen delivery to muscles.
    - Sources: Meat, fish, eggs, dairy products, legumes, and leafy green vegetables.

Minerals

1. Magnesium
    - Function: Involved in muscle contraction and relaxation, energy production, and protein synthesis.
    - Sources: Leafy green vegetables, nuts, seeds, whole grains, and supplements.
2. Calcium
    - Function: Crucial for muscle contraction and nerve signaling.
    - Sources: Dairy products, fortified plant-based milks, leafy green vegetables, and supplements.
3. Potassium

- Function: Electrolyte that helps
    maintain proper muscle function
    and prevents cramps.
  - Sources: Bananas, sweet
    potatoes, avocados, spinach, and
    tomatoes.
4. Zinc
  - Function: Supports protein
    synthesis and muscle repair.
  - Sources: Meat, shellfish, legumes,
    seeds, and nuts.

Herbs

1. Turmeric (Curcuma longa)
   - Function: Contains curcumin,
     which has anti-inflammatory and
     antioxidant properties that can
     reduce muscle soreness and
     enhance recovery.
   - Uses: Fresh root, powder,
     capsules, and teas.
2. Ashwagandha (Withania somnifera)
   - Function: Adaptogen that helps
     improve muscle strength, reduce
     muscle damage, and support
     recovery.
   - Uses: Powder, capsules, tinctures.

3. Ginger (Zingiber officinale)
   - Function: Anti-inflammatory properties that can help reduce muscle pain and soreness.
   - Uses: Fresh root, dried, capsules, and teas.
4. Ginseng (Panax ginseng)
   - Function: Enhances physical performance, reduces fatigue, and supports muscle recovery.
   - Uses: Capsules, extracts, and teas.
5. Boswellia (Boswellia serrata)
   - Function: Anti-inflammatory properties that help reduce muscle inflammation and pain.
   - Uses: Capsules, extracts, and topical creams.

Nutritional Support

1. Protein
   - Function: Essential for muscle repair and growth.
   - Sources: Lean meats, fish, eggs, dairy, legumes, nuts, and seeds.
2. Omega-3 Fatty Acids

- Function: Anti-inflammatory
    properties that aid in muscle
    recovery and reduce muscle
    soreness.
  - Sources: Fatty fish, flaxseeds,
    chia seeds, walnuts, and
    supplements.

3. Collagen
  - Function: Supports the structure
    of muscles and connective
    tissues, aiding in repair and
    recovery.
  - Sources: Bone broth, collagen
    supplements, and gelatin.

Cardiac Muscles

Structure of Cardiac Muscles

- Cardiomyocytes: Cardiac muscle cells, or cardiomyocytes, are branched, cylindrical cells with a single central nucleus. They are shorter in length compared to skeletal muscle fibers.
- Striations: Cardiac muscles have a striated appearance due to the arrangement of actin and myosin filaments in sarcomeres.
- Intercalated Discs: Specialized structures that connect cardiomyocytes. They contain:
    - Gap Junctions: Allow direct passage of ions and electrical impulses between cells, enabling synchronized contraction.
    - Desmosomes: Provide mechanical strength, preventing cells from being pulled apart during contraction.
- Sarcoplasmic Reticulum (SR) and T-Tubules:
    - SR: Stores calcium ions essential for muscle contraction.

- T-Tubules: Invaginations of the sarcolemma (cell membrane) that help transmit action potentials into the cell's interior.
- Mitochondria: High density of mitochondria provides the energy needed for continuous contraction through aerobic respiration.

Function of Cardiac Muscles

- Pumping Blood: Cardiac muscles contract rhythmically and continuously to pump blood throughout the body.
- Control: Involuntary control by the autonomic nervous system.
- Electrical Conduction System: Coordinates the contraction of the heart, ensuring efficient blood flow. Components include the sinoatrial (SA) node, atrioventricular (AV) node, bundle of His, bundle branches, and Purkinje fibers.
- Contractility: Involves the sliding filament theory where actin and myosin filaments slide past each other to produce contraction.

- Automaticity: The ability to generate spontaneous electrical activity. The SA node serves as the natural pacemaker of the heart.
- Rhythmicity: The ability to contract in a regular and rhythmic manner.
- Excitability: The ability to respond to electrical stimuli.
- Conductivity: The ability to conduct electrical impulses rapidly between cells.

Herbs, Minerals, Vitamins, and Supplements for Cardiac Muscle Health

Maintaining healthy cardiac muscles involves a combination of essential nutrients and lifestyle practices. Here are specific herbs, minerals, vitamins, and supplements that support the health and function of the cardiac muscles:

Vitamins

1. Vitamin D

- Function: Enhances calcium
  absorption, which is crucial for
  muscle contraction and overall
  heart health.
- Sources: Sunlight, fortified dairy
  products, fatty fish (salmon,
  mackerel), supplements.

2. Vitamin C
    - Function: Antioxidant that
      protects heart cells from oxidative
      stress and supports collagen
      synthesis.
    - Sources: Citrus fruits,
      strawberries, bell peppers,
      broccoli, supplements.

3. Vitamin E
    - Function: Antioxidant that helps
      prevent oxidative damage to
      cardiac tissues.
    - Sources: Nuts, seeds, spinach,
      vegetable oils.

4. B Vitamins (B6, B12, Folate)
    - Function: Support energy
      production and red blood cell
      formation, essential for oxygen
      delivery to the heart.
    - Sources: Meat, fish, eggs, dairy
      products, legumes, leafy green
      vegetables.

Minerals

1. Magnesium
   - Function: Important for maintaining a normal heart rhythm and muscle function.
   - Sources: Leafy green vegetables, nuts, seeds, whole grains, supplements.
2. Calcium
   - Function: Crucial for muscle contraction and nerve signaling in the heart.
   - Sources: Dairy products, fortified plant-based milks, leafy green vegetables, supplements.
3. Potassium
   - Function: Essential for maintaining proper electrical conductivity in the heart.
   - Sources: Bananas, sweet potatoes, avocados, spinach, tomatoes.
4. Zinc
   - Function: Supports protein synthesis and muscle repair, including cardiac muscle.
   - Sources: Meat, shellfish, legumes, seeds, nuts.

Herbs

1. Hawthorn (Crataegus spp.)
    - Function: Supports cardiovascular health by improving blood flow and reducing blood pressure.
    - Uses: Berries, leaves, and flowers used in teas, capsules, and extracts.
2. Garlic (Allium sativum)
    - Function: Reduces blood pressure and cholesterol levels, supporting overall heart health.
    - Uses: Fresh cloves, capsules, extracts.
3. Turmeric (Curcuma longa)
    - Function: Contains curcumin, which has anti-inflammatory and antioxidant properties beneficial for heart health.
    - Uses: Fresh root, powder, capsules, teas.
4. Arjuna (Terminalia arjuna)
    - Function: Traditionally used in Ayurvedic medicine to support heart function and improve cardiovascular health.
    - Uses: Bark used in teas, capsules, extracts.

5. Ginseng (Panax ginseng)
   - Function: Enhances physical performance, reduces fatigue, and supports cardiovascular health.
   - Uses: Capsules, extracts, teas.

Supplements

1. Coenzyme Q10 (CoQ10)
   - Function: Antioxidant that supports mitochondrial function and energy production in cardiac cells.
   - Sources: Meat, fish, whole grains, supplements.
2. Omega-3 Fatty Acids
   - Function: Anti-inflammatory properties that support heart health and reduce the risk of arrhythmias.
   - Sources: Fatty fish (salmon, mackerel), flaxseeds, chia seeds, walnuts, supplements.
3. L-Carnitine
   - Function: Plays a crucial role in energy production by

transporting fatty acids into the mitochondria.
- Sources: Meat, fish, poultry, dairy products, supplements.

4. Resveratrol
- Function: Antioxidant that supports heart health by reducing inflammation and oxidative stress.
- Sources: Red wine, grapes, berries, supplements.

5. Taurine
- Function: Supports heart function by regulating calcium levels and maintaining electrolyte balance.
- Sources: Meat, fish, dairy products, supplements.

Lifestyle Practices

1. Regular Exercise
- Importance: Strengthens the heart muscle, improves circulation, and reduces the risk of cardiovascular disease.

- Types: Aerobic exercises like walking, running, cycling, and swimming.

2. Healthy Diet
    - Focus: A diet rich in fruits, vegetables, whole grains, lean proteins, and healthy fats supports heart health.
    - Avoid: Excessive intake of processed foods, saturated fats, and high-sodium foods.

3. Stress Management
    - Techniques: Meditation, yoga, deep breathing exercises, and other relaxation techniques to reduce stress and its impact on heart health.

4. Adequate Sleep
    - Importance: Essential for overall health and heart function.
    - Advice: Aim for 7-9 hours of quality sleep per night.

5. Avoid Smoking and Limit Alcohol
    - Impact: Smoking and excessive alcohol consumption can have detrimental effects on heart health.

Smooth Muscles

Structure of Smooth Muscles

- Cell Shape and Size:
    - Spindle-shaped: Smooth muscle cells are elongated, spindle-shaped with tapered ends.
    - Single Nucleus: Each cell contains a single, centrally located nucleus.
    - Size: Smaller than skeletal muscle fibers, typically 20-200 micrometers in length.
- Non-Striated Appearance:
    - Unlike skeletal and cardiac muscles, smooth muscles lack striations due to the irregular arrangement of actin and myosin filaments.
- Cellular Components:
    - Actin and Myosin Filaments: Though present, these filaments are arranged irregularly, contributing to the muscle's non-striated appearance.

- Dense Bodies: Analogous to Z-discs in skeletal muscle, they anchor actin filaments and help transmit the force of contraction.
- Intermediate Filaments: Provide structural support and stability to the cells.

Function of Smooth Muscles

- Involuntary Control:
    - Operate under the control of the autonomic nervous system (ANS) and hormones.
    - Function independently of conscious thought.
- Slow, Sustained Contractions:
    - Can maintain contractions for extended periods without fatigue, suitable for roles requiring constant muscle tone and sustained contraction.
- Locations and Specific Functions:
    - Blood Vessels: Regulate blood flow and pressure by contracting and relaxing the vessel walls (vasoconstriction and vasodilation).

- Digestive Tract: Propel food and waste through the gastrointestinal tract via peristalsis.
- Respiratory Tract: Control the diameter of airways.
- Urinary System: Facilitate the movement of urine from the kidneys to the bladder and out of the body.
- Reproductive System: Involved in various functions such as the movement of sperm, contraction of the uterus during childbirth, and control of reproductive organ functions.

Characteristics of Smooth Muscles

- Plasticity:
    - Ability to stretch and adapt to new lengths while maintaining the ability to contract.
- Excitability:
    - Respond to stimuli such as hormones, neural inputs, and changes in local chemical environment.

- Automaticity:
    - Some smooth muscles, like those in the gastrointestinal tract, can generate their own rhythmic contractions through pacemaker cells.
- Connectivity:
    - Cells are often connected by gap junctions, allowing for coordinated contractions as a single unit, especially in visceral smooth muscle.

Types of Smooth Muscle

- Single-Unit (Visceral) Smooth Muscle:
    - Found in the walls of hollow organs (e.g., intestines, bladder).
    - Cells contract together as a single unit due to the presence of gap junctions.
- Multi-Unit Smooth Muscle:
    - Found in locations such as the iris of the eye, arrector pili muscles in the skin, and large airways of the lungs.
    - Cells contract independently, allowing for more precise control.

Herbs, Minerals, Vitamins, and Supplements for Smooth Muscle Health

Supporting, maintaining, and healing smooth muscles requires a combination of essential nutrients and beneficial herbs. Here are some key vitamins, minerals, herbs, and supplements that contribute to the health and function of smooth muscles:

Vitamins

1. Vitamin C
   - Function: Essential for collagen synthesis, which is important for the structural integrity of smooth muscles.
   - Sources: Citrus fruits, strawberries, bell peppers, broccoli, kiwi, supplements.
2. Vitamin E
   - Function: Acts as an antioxidant, protecting smooth muscle cells from oxidative stress and damage.
   - Sources: Nuts, seeds, spinach, vegetable oils, supplements.

3. Vitamin D
   - Function: Plays a role in calcium absorption and muscle function.
   - Sources: Sunlight, fortified dairy products, fatty fish (salmon, mackerel), supplements.
4. B Vitamins (B1, B6, B12)
   - Function: Support energy production and proper nerve function, which are essential for smooth muscle activity.
   - Sources: Meat, fish, eggs, dairy products, whole grains, legumes, leafy green vegetables, supplements.

Minerals

1. Magnesium
   - Function: Crucial for muscle relaxation and preventing cramps in smooth muscles.
   - Sources: Leafy green vegetables, nuts, seeds, whole grains, legumes, supplements.
2. Calcium

- Function: Essential for muscle contraction and proper signaling in smooth muscles.
- Sources: Dairy products, fortified plant-based milks, leafy green vegetables, supplements.

3. Potassium
    - Function: Important for maintaining electrolyte balance and smooth muscle function.
    - Sources: Bananas, sweet potatoes, avocados, spinach, tomatoes, supplements.

4. Zinc
    - Function: Supports protein synthesis and muscle repair, including smooth muscle.
    - Sources: Meat, shellfish, legumes, seeds, nuts, supplements.

Herbs

1. Peppermint (Mentha piperita)
    - Function: Relieves smooth muscle spasms and cramps, especially in the digestive tract.
    - Uses: Teas, essential oils, capsules.

2. Chamomile (Matricaria chamomilla)
    - Function: Anti-inflammatory and antispasmodic properties that soothe smooth muscle tension.
    - Uses: Teas, extracts, capsules.
3. Ginger (Zingiber officinale)
    - Function: Reduces inflammation and can help soothe digestive smooth muscle discomfort.
    - Uses: Fresh root, teas, capsules, extracts.
4. Turmeric (Curcuma longa)
    - Function: Contains curcumin, which has anti-inflammatory and muscle-relaxing properties.
    - Uses: Fresh root, powder, capsules, extracts.
5. Licorice (Glycyrrhiza glabra)
    - Function: Soothes mucous membranes and smooth muscle tissues, especially in the digestive tract.
    - Uses: Teas, extracts, capsules.

Supplements

1. Omega-3 Fatty Acids

- Function: Anti-inflammatory
  properties that support muscle
  health and reduce the risk of
  muscle spasms.
- Sources: Fatty fish (salmon,
  mackerel), flaxseeds, chia seeds,
  walnuts, supplements.

2. L-Arginine
   - Function: An amino acid that
     helps improve blood flow and can
     aid in smooth muscle relaxation.
   - Sources: Meat, poultry, dairy
     products, nuts, seeds,
     supplements.

3. Coenzyme Q10 (CoQ10)
   - Function: Antioxidant that
     supports energy production in
     muscle cells.
   - Sources: Meat, fish, whole grains,
     supplements.

4. Probiotics
   - Function: Supports a healthy
     digestive system, which relies
     heavily on smooth muscle
     function.
   - Sources: Yogurt, kefir, fermented
     foods, supplements.

5. Taurine

- Function: Supports muscle function and helps regulate calcium levels in cells.
- Sources: Meat, fish, dairy products, supplements.

Type I (Slow-Twitch) Muscle Fibers

Structure of Type I Muscle Fibers

- Size and Shape:
    - Smaller in diameter compared to Type II (fast-twitch) fibers.
    - Red in color due to high myoglobin content.
- Mitochondria:
    - High density of mitochondria, which are the powerhouses of the cell, providing a continuous supply of ATP through aerobic respiration.
- Capillary Supply:
    - Rich capillary network, ensuring an ample supply of oxygen and nutrients and the efficient removal of waste products.
- Myoglobin Content:
    - High myoglobin content, which stores oxygen and facilitates oxygen transport within the muscle cell.

Function of Type I Muscle Fibers

- Endurance Activities:
  - Specialized for prolonged, sustained activities that require endurance rather than quick bursts of power.
  - Common in muscles involved in posture maintenance and endurance sports such as marathon running, cycling, and swimming.
- Aerobic Metabolism:
  - Rely predominantly on aerobic metabolism (oxidative phosphorylation) for ATP production, which is efficient and sustainable over long periods.
- Fatigue Resistance:
  - Highly resistant to fatigue, allowing them to sustain activity for extended periods without tiring.

Characteristics of Type I Muscle Fibers

- Contraction Speed:

- Slow contraction speed compared to fast-twitch fibers.
  - Slow myosin ATPase activity, resulting in a slower rate of cross-bridge cycling.
- Force Production:
  - Lower force production compared to fast-twitch fibers, but capable of maintaining force output over long durations.
- Energy Source:
  - Primarily use fats and carbohydrates as energy sources, with a high reliance on oxidative phosphorylation.
- Adaptability:
  - Highly adaptable to endurance training, leading to increased mitochondrial density, capillary supply, and oxidative enzymes.

Distribution in the Body

- Postural Muscles:
  - Abundant in muscles that maintain posture and support the body against gravity, such as the

muscles of the lower back and legs.
- Endurance Athletes:
  - Higher proportion in the muscles of endurance athletes, who perform activities that require prolonged aerobic capacity.

Type I (slow-twitch) muscle fibers are specialized for endurance and sustained activities, characterized by their slow contraction speed, high fatigue resistance, and reliance on aerobic metabolism. They have a rich supply of mitochondria, capillaries, and myoglobin, making them efficient at using oxygen to produce ATP over long periods. These fibers are essential for maintaining posture and performing endurance activities, and they adapt well to endurance training, enhancing their capacity for sustained performance.

Herbs, Minerals, Vitamins, and Supplements for Restoring Type I (Slow-Twitch) Muscle Fibers

Maintaining and restoring Type I muscle fibers, which are essential for endurance and sustained activities, requires specific nutrients and herbs. Here are some key vitamins, minerals, herbs, and supplements that support the health and function of slow-twitch muscle fibers:

Vitamins

1. Vitamin D
    - Function: Enhances calcium absorption and plays a role in muscle function and strength.
    - Sources: Sunlight, fortified dairy products, fatty fish (salmon, mackerel), supplements.
2. Vitamin B12
    - Function: Supports red blood cell formation and oxygen transport, crucial for muscle endurance.

- Sources: Meat, fish, eggs, dairy products, fortified cereals, supplements.

3. Vitamin C
   - Function: Antioxidant that helps with collagen synthesis, important for muscle tissue repair and health.
   - Sources: Citrus fruits, strawberries, bell peppers, broccoli, kiwi, supplements.
4. Vitamin E
   - Function: Protects muscle cells from oxidative damage and supports overall muscle health.
   - Sources: Nuts, seeds, spinach, vegetable oils, supplements.

Minerals

1. Magnesium
   - Function: Vital for muscle relaxation and preventing cramps; involved in energy production.
   - Sources: Leafy green vegetables, nuts, seeds, whole grains, legumes, supplements.

2. Calcium
   - Function: Essential for muscle contraction and signaling within muscle cells.
   - Sources: Dairy products, fortified plant-based milks, leafy green vegetables, supplements.
3. Iron
   - Function: Important for oxygen transport in the blood, crucial for endurance and muscle performance.
   - Sources: Red meat, poultry, fish, lentils, beans, spinach, supplements.
4. Potassium
   - Function: Helps maintain electrolyte balance and supports proper muscle function.
   - Sources: Bananas, sweet potatoes, avocados, spinach, tomatoes, supplements.

Herbs

1. Ashwagandha (Withania somnifera)
   - Function: Adaptogen that helps increase endurance, reduce

fatigue, and improve muscle recovery.

- Uses: Capsules, extracts, teas.

2. Rhodiola (Rhodiola rosea)
   - Function: Improves endurance and reduces fatigue by enhancing oxygen utilization.
   - Uses: Capsules, extracts, teas.
3. Ginseng (Panax ginseng)
   - Function: Enhances physical performance and reduces fatigue, supporting muscle endurance.
   - Uses: Capsules, extracts, teas.
4. Cordyceps (Cordyceps sinensis)
   - Function: Increases energy production and endurance by improving oxygen utilization.
   - Uses: Capsules, powders, extracts.
5. Turmeric (Curcuma longa)
   - Function: Contains curcumin, which has anti-inflammatory properties that support muscle recovery.
   - Uses: Fresh root, powder, capsules, extracts.

Supplements

1. Omega-3 Fatty Acids
   - Function: Reduce inflammation and support muscle recovery and endurance.
   - Sources: Fish oil, flaxseed oil, chia seeds, walnuts, supplements.
2. Creatine Monohydrate
   - Function: Enhances energy production and improves muscle endurance and recovery.
   - Sources: Supplements.
3. Beta-Alanine
   - Function: Helps buffer acid in muscles, improving endurance and reducing fatigue.
   - Sources: Supplements.
4. L-Carnitine
   - Function: Supports fat metabolism and energy production in muscle cells.
   - Sources: Meat, fish, poultry, dairy products, supplements.
5. Branched-Chain Amino Acids (BCAAs)

- Function: Support muscle protein synthesis and reduce muscle breakdown during prolonged exercise.
- Sources: Supplements.

Type IIa (Fast-Twitch Oxidative) Muscle Fibers

Structure of Type IIa Muscle Fibers

- Size and Shape:
    - Larger in diameter than Type I (slow-twitch) fibers but smaller than Type IIb (fast-twitch glycolytic) fibers.
    - Red to pink in color due to moderate myoglobin content.
- Mitochondria:
    - Moderate to high density of mitochondria, which support both aerobic and anaerobic metabolism.
- Capillary Supply:
    - Well-developed capillary network, though not as extensive as in Type I fibers, ensuring a good supply of oxygen and nutrients.
- Myoglobin Content:
    - Moderate myoglobin content, providing a balance between

oxygen storage and transport within the muscle cell.

Function of Type IIa Muscle Fibers

- Versatility in Activities:
    - Specialized for activities requiring both endurance and strength.
    - Used in sports and activities that involve moderate-duration, high-intensity efforts, such as middle-distance running, swimming, and cycling.
- Aerobic and Anaerobic Metabolism:
    - Can generate ATP through both oxidative (aerobic) and glycolytic (anaerobic) pathways, making them versatile in energy production.
- Moderate Fatigue Resistance:
    - More resistant to fatigue than Type IIb fibers but less so than Type I fibers.

Characteristics of Type IIa Muscle Fibers

- Contraction Speed:
    - Faster contraction speed compared to Type I fibers.
    - Intermediate myosin ATPase activity, resulting in a faster rate of cross-bridge cycling than Type I fibers.
- Force Production:
    - Higher force production than Type I fibers but less than Type IIb fibers.
- Energy Source:
    - Utilize both carbohydrates and fats for energy, with a higher reliance on glycolysis during high-intensity activities.
- Adaptability:
    - Adapt well to both endurance and strength training, leading to improvements in both aerobic capacity and muscle strength.

Distribution in the Body

- Mixed Muscles:

- - Abundant in muscles that require a combination of strength and endurance, such as the muscles used in running, cycling, and swimming.
  - Athletes:
    - Higher proportion in the muscles of athletes who engage in sports that require a balance of endurance and power.

Type IIa (fast-twitch oxidative) muscle fibers are specialized for activities that require both endurance and strength. They are characterized by their moderate contraction speed, intermediate fatigue resistance, and ability to generate ATP through both aerobic and anaerobic metabolism. These fibers have a well-developed capillary network and moderate myoglobin content, making them versatile for activities that involve sustained, high-intensity efforts. Type IIa fibers adapt well to both endurance and strength training, enhancing their capacity for both aerobic and anaerobic performance.

Herbs, Vitamins, Minerals, and Supplements for Type IIa (Fast-Twitch Oxidative) Muscle Fibers

Supporting and maintaining Type IIa muscle fibers, which are essential for activities requiring both endurance and strength, involves specific nutrients and herbs. Here are some key vitamins, minerals, herbs, and supplements that contribute to the health and function of fast-twitch oxidative muscle fibers:

Vitamins

1. Vitamin B6 (Pyridoxine)
   - Function: Important for protein metabolism and muscle growth.
   - Sources: Poultry, fish, potatoes, chickpeas, bananas, supplements.
2. Vitamin B12 (Cobalamin)
   - Function: Supports red blood cell formation and oxygen transport, crucial for muscle endurance and performance.

- Sources: Meat, fish, dairy products, eggs, fortified cereals, supplements.

3. Vitamin D
   - Function: Enhances calcium absorption and plays a role in muscle function and strength.
   - Sources: Sunlight, fortified dairy products, fatty fish, supplements.
4. Vitamin E
   - Function: Acts as an antioxidant, protecting muscle cells from oxidative damage.
   - Sources: Nuts, seeds, spinach, vegetable oils, supplements.

Minerals

1. Magnesium
   - Function: Essential for muscle relaxation and energy production, helps prevent cramps and muscle fatigue.
   - Sources: Leafy green vegetables, nuts, seeds, whole grains, legumes, supplements.
2. Calcium

- Function: Vital for muscle
  contraction and signaling within
  muscle cells.
- Sources: Dairy products, fortified
  plant-based milks, leafy green
  vegetables, supplements.

3. Iron
   - Function: Important for oxygen
     transport in the blood, essential
     for muscle performance and
     endurance.
   - Sources: Red meat, poultry, fish,
     lentils, beans, spinach,
     supplements.

4. Zinc
   - Function: Supports protein
     synthesis and muscle repair.
   - Sources: Meat, shellfish, legumes,
     seeds, nuts, supplements.

Herbs

1. Ginseng (Panax ginseng)
   - Function: Enhances physical
     performance and reduces fatigue,
     supporting muscle endurance
     and strength.
   - Uses: Capsules, extracts, teas.

2. Rhodiola (Rhodiola rosea)
    - Function: Improves endurance and reduces fatigue by enhancing oxygen utilization.
    - Uses: Capsules, extracts, teas.
3. Ashwagandha (Withania somnifera)
    - Function: Adaptogen that helps increase endurance, reduce fatigue, and improve muscle recovery.
    - Uses: Capsules, extracts, teas.
4. Cordyceps (Cordyceps sinensis)
    - Function: Increases energy production and endurance by improving oxygen utilization.
    - Uses: Capsules, powders, extracts.
5. Turmeric (Curcuma longa)
    - Function: Contains curcumin, which has anti-inflammatory properties that support muscle recovery.
    - Uses: Fresh root, powder, capsules, extracts.

Supplements

1. Creatine Monohydrate

- Function: Enhances energy production, improves muscle strength, and supports muscle endurance.
    - Sources: Supplements.
2. Beta-Alanine
    - Function: Helps buffer acid in muscles, improving endurance and reducing fatigue.
    - Sources: Supplements.
3. L-Carnitine
    - Function: Supports fat metabolism and energy production in muscle cells.
    - Sources: Meat, fish, poultry, dairy products, supplements.
4. Branched-Chain Amino Acids (BCAAs)
    - Function: Support muscle protein synthesis and reduce muscle breakdown during exercise.
    - Sources: Supplements.
5. Omega-3 Fatty Acids
    - Function: Reduce inflammation and support muscle recovery and endurance.
    - Sources: Fish oil, flaxseed oil, chia seeds, walnuts, supplements.
6. Coenzyme Q10 (CoQ10)

- Function: Antioxidant that
  supports energy production in
  muscle cells.
- Sources: Meat, fish, whole grains,
  supplements.

7. Nitric Oxide Boosters (e.g., L-Arginine,
L-Citrulline)

- Function: Improve blood flow to
  muscles, enhancing oxygen
  delivery and muscle performance.
- Sources: Supplements.

Type IIb (Fast-Twitch Glycolytic) Muscle Fibers

Structure of Type IIb Muscle Fibers

- Size and Shape:
    - Largest in diameter among the muscle fiber types.
    - Pale or white in color due to low myoglobin content.
- Mitochondria:
    - Low density of mitochondria compared to Type I and Type IIa fibers, relying primarily on anaerobic metabolism.
- Capillary Supply:
    - Sparse capillary network, reflecting their lower reliance on oxygen for energy production.
- Myoglobin Content:
    - Low myoglobin content, as they are not primarily dependent on oxygen for energy.

Function of Type IIb Muscle Fibers

- Quick, Powerful Movements:
    - Specialized for short bursts of power and strength rather than endurance.
    - Activated during high-intensity, short-duration activities like sprinting, weightlifting, and jumping.
- Anaerobic Metabolism:
    - Generate ATP predominantly through anaerobic glycolysis, allowing for rapid energy production without the need for oxygen.
- Fatigue Susceptibility:
    - Fatigue quickly due to the accumulation of lactic acid and depletion of energy reserves.

Characteristics of Type IIb Muscle Fibers

- Contraction Speed:
    - Fastest contraction speed among the muscle fiber types.

- High myosin ATPase activity,
    leading to rapid cross-bridge
    cycling.
- Force Production:
  - Highest force production
    compared to Type I and Type IIa
    fibers.
- Energy Source:
  - Primarily rely on glycogen stored
    within the muscle for energy
    through glycolysis.
  - Less efficient at using fats and
    other fuel sources.
- Adaptability:
  - Respond well to strength and
    power training, increasing muscle
    size (hypertrophy) and strength.

Distribution in the Body

- Power Muscles:
  - Found in greater abundance in
    muscles used for powerful,
    explosive movements such as the
    quadriceps, hamstrings, and
    muscles of the upper arms.
- Athletes:

- Higher proportion in the muscles of athletes who participate in sports requiring quick bursts of strength and speed, such as sprinters, weightlifters, and football players.

Type IIb (fast-twitch glycolytic) muscle fibers are specialized for quick, powerful movements and are characterized by their large diameter, fast contraction speed, high force production, and reliance on anaerobic metabolism. These fibers have a low density of mitochondria and capillaries, and they fatigue quickly due to the accumulation of lactic acid. Type IIb fibers are crucial for high-intensity, short-duration activities and respond well to strength and power training, making them essential for sports and activities that require rapid, explosive power.

Herbs, Vitamins, Minerals, and Supplements for Type IIb (Fast-Twitch Glycolytic) Muscle Fibers

Supporting and maintaining Type IIb muscle fibers, which are essential for quick, powerful movements, requires specific nutrients and herbs. Here are some key vitamins, minerals, herbs, and supplements that contribute to the health and function of fast-twitch glycolytic muscle fibers:

Vitamins

1. Vitamin B6 (Pyridoxine)
    - Function: Important for protein metabolism and muscle growth.
    - Sources: Poultry, fish, potatoes, chickpeas, bananas, supplements.
2. Vitamin B12 (Cobalamin)
    - Function: Supports red blood cell formation and oxygen transport, crucial for muscle performance.
    - Sources: Meat, fish, dairy products, eggs, fortified cereals, supplements.

3. Vitamin D
   - Function: Enhances calcium absorption and plays a role in muscle function and strength.
   - Sources: Sunlight, fortified dairy products, fatty fish, supplements.
4. Vitamin C
   - Function: Antioxidant that helps with collagen synthesis, important for muscle tissue repair.
   - Sources: Citrus fruits, strawberries, bell peppers, broccoli, kiwi, supplements.

Minerals

1. Magnesium
   - Function: Essential for muscle relaxation and energy production, helps prevent cramps and muscle fatigue.
   - Sources: Leafy green vegetables, nuts, seeds, whole grains, legumes, supplements.
2. Calcium

- Function: Vital for muscle contraction and signaling within muscle cells.
    - Sources: Dairy products, fortified plant-based milks, leafy green vegetables, supplements.
3. Zinc
    - Function: Supports protein synthesis and muscle repair.
    - Sources: Meat, shellfish, legumes, seeds, nuts, supplements.
4. Phosphorus
    - Function: Important for energy production and muscle contraction.
    - Sources: Meat, poultry, fish, dairy products, nuts, seeds, supplements.

Herbs

1. Ginseng (Panax ginseng)
    - Function: Enhances physical performance and reduces fatigue, supporting muscle strength and power.
    - Uses: Capsules, extracts, teas.
2. Rhodiola (Rhodiola rosea)

- Function: Improves endurance and reduces fatigue by enhancing oxygen utilization and energy production.
- Uses: Capsules, extracts, teas.

3. Ashwagandha (Withania somnifera)
   - Function: Adaptogen that helps increase strength, reduce fatigue, and improve muscle recovery.
   - Uses: Capsules, extracts, teas.
4. Eleuthero (Eleutherococcus senticosus)
   - Function: Increases stamina and reduces fatigue, supporting high-intensity muscle performance.
   - Uses: Capsules, extracts, teas.
5. Tribulus Terrestris
   - Function: May support testosterone levels, enhancing muscle strength and performance.
   - Uses: Capsules, extracts, powders.

Supplements

1. Creatine Monohydrate

- Function: Enhances ATP production, improves muscle strength, power, and performance during high-intensity activities.
    - Sources: Supplements.
2. Beta-Alanine
    - Function: Helps buffer acid in muscles, improving endurance and reducing fatigue during high-intensity activities.
    - Sources: Supplements.
3. L-Arginine
    - Function: Precursor to nitric oxide, which improves blood flow to muscles, enhancing oxygen delivery and muscle performance.
    - Sources: Supplements.
4. Branched-Chain Amino Acids (BCAAs)
    - Function: Support muscle protein synthesis and reduce muscle breakdown during high-intensity exercise.
    - Sources: Supplements.
5. HMB (Beta-Hydroxy Beta-Methylbutyrate)
    - Function: Supports muscle protein synthesis and reduces muscle breakdown.

- Sources: Supplements.
6. Caffeine
    - Function: Enhances alertness and reduces perceived effort during high-intensity activities, improving performance.
    - Sources: Coffee, tea, supplements.
7. Nitric Oxide Boosters (e.g., L-Citrulline)
    - Function: Improve blood flow to muscles, enhancing oxygen and nutrient delivery.
    - Sources: Supplements.
8. Taurine
    - Function: Supports muscle contraction and reduces muscle damage during high-intensity exercise.
    - Sources: Meat, fish, dairy products, supplements.

Myofibrils: Structure and Function

Definition and Overview

Myofibrils are the basic rod-like units of a muscle cell (muscle fiber). They are essential for muscle contraction and are composed of repeating sections called sarcomeres, which are the functional units of muscle fibers.

Structure of Myofibrils

- Sarcomeres:
    - The smallest contractile units of myofibrils.
    - Bounded by Z-discs (Z-lines) which anchor the actin filaments.
    - Contain thick (myosin) and thin (actin) filaments that slide past each other during muscle contraction.
- Myofilaments:
    - Thick Filaments:
        - Composed primarily of the protein myosin.

- Myosin molecules have
  heads that bind to actin
  during contraction.
- Thin Filaments:
  - Composed primarily of the
    protein actin.
  - Also contain tropomyosin
    and troponin, regulatory
    proteins that control the
    interaction of actin and
    myosin.
- Banding Pattern:
  - A-Band: The dark area where
    thick and thin filaments overlap.
  - I-Band: The light area containing
    only thin filaments.
  - H-Zone: The central part of the
    A-Band where only thick
    filaments are present.
  - M-Line: The middle line within
    the H-Zone that holds the thick
    filaments together.

Function of Myofibrils

- Muscle Contraction:
  - Sliding Filament Theory:
    Explains how muscles contract.

Myosin heads bind to actin filaments forming cross-bridges and then pull the actin filaments toward the center of the sarcomere, shortening the muscle.

- ATP Role: ATP provides the energy for the myosin heads to attach, pivot, and detach from the actin filaments.

- Force Generation:
    - The interaction between myosin and actin generates force and movement.
    - The number of myofibrils within a muscle fiber determines its strength; more myofibrils mean a stronger muscle.

Myofibril Development and Growth

- Hypertrophy:
    - Increase in the size of muscle fibers due to an increase in the size and number of myofibrils.
    - Common in response to resistance training and strength training.

- Hyperplasia:
    - Increase in the number of muscle fibers, which may contribute to muscle growth but is less common than hypertrophy.

Disorders Related to Myofibrils

- Muscular Dystrophy:
    - A group of genetic disorders causing muscle weakness and degeneration due to defects in muscle proteins, including those in myofibrils.
- Myopathies:
    - A variety of diseases affecting muscle function, often linked to abnormalities in myofibril structure or function.

Myofibrils are the fundamental components of muscle fibers responsible for muscle contraction. They are composed of sarcomeres, which contain actin and myosin filaments that slide past each other to produce movement. The structure and function of myofibrils are crucial for force generation and muscle strength. Understanding myofibrils is essential for comprehending how muscles work, how they grow in response to exercise, and how certain muscle diseases affect their function.

Herbs, Vitamins, Minerals, and Supplements for Supporting Myofibrils

Supporting the health and function of myofibrils is essential for muscle strength, repair, and overall performance. Here are some key nutrients, herbs, and supplements that contribute to the maintenance and enhancement of myofibrils:

Vitamins

1. Vitamin D
   - Function: Enhances calcium absorption, essential for muscle contraction and strength.

- Sources: Sunlight, fortified dairy products, fatty fish, supplements.

2. Vitamin E
   - Function: Acts as an antioxidant, protecting muscle cells from oxidative stress and damage.
   - Sources: Nuts, seeds, spinach, vegetable oils, supplements.

3. Vitamin C
   - Function: Essential for collagen synthesis, important for muscle repair and connective tissue health.
   - Sources: Citrus fruits, strawberries, bell peppers, broccoli, kiwi, supplements.

4. Vitamin B6 (Pyridoxine)
   - Function: Important for protein metabolism and muscle growth.
   - Sources: Poultry, fish, potatoes, chickpeas, bananas, supplements.

5. Vitamin B12 (Cobalamin)
   - Function: Supports red blood cell formation and oxygen transport, crucial for muscle performance.
   - Sources: Meat, fish, dairy products, eggs, fortified cereals, supplements.

Minerals

1. Magnesium
    - Function: Essential for muscle relaxation and energy production, helps prevent cramps and muscle fatigue.
    - Sources: Leafy green vegetables, nuts, seeds, whole grains, legumes, supplements.
2. Calcium
    - Function: Vital for muscle contraction and signaling within muscle cells.
    - Sources: Dairy products, fortified plant-based milks, leafy green vegetables, supplements.
3. Zinc
    - Function: Supports protein synthesis and muscle repair.
    - Sources: Meat, shellfish, legumes, seeds, nuts, supplements.
4. Iron
    - Function: Important for oxygen transport in the blood, essential for muscle performance and endurance.
    - Sources: Red meat, poultry, fish, lentils, beans, spinach, supplements.

Herbs

1. Ashwagandha (Withania somnifera)
    - Function: Adaptogen that helps increase strength, reduce fatigue, and improve muscle recovery.
    - Uses: Capsules, extracts, teas.
2. Ginseng (Panax ginseng)
    - Function: Enhances physical performance and reduces fatigue, supporting muscle strength and endurance.
    - Uses: Capsules, extracts, teas.
3. Turmeric (Curcuma longa)
    - Function: Contains curcumin, which has anti-inflammatory properties that support muscle recovery.
    - Uses: Fresh root, powder, capsules, extracts.
4. Rhodiola (Rhodiola rosea)
    - Function: Improves endurance and reduces fatigue by enhancing oxygen utilization.
    - Uses: Capsules, extracts, teas.
5. Eleuthero (Eleutherococcus senticosus)
    - Function: Increases stamina and reduces fatigue, supporting high-intensity muscle performance.

- Uses: Capsules, extracts, teas.

Supplements

1. Creatine Monohydrate
   - Function: Enhances ATP production, improves muscle strength, power, and performance during high-intensity activities.
   - Sources: Supplements.
2. Beta-Alanine
   - Function: Helps buffer acid in muscles, improving endurance and reducing fatigue during high-intensity activities.
   - Sources: Supplements.
3. L-Arginine
   - Function: Precursor to nitric oxide, which improves blood flow to muscles, enhancing oxygen delivery and muscle performance.
   - Sources: Supplements.
4. Branched-Chain Amino Acids (BCAAs)
   - Function: Support muscle protein synthesis and reduce muscle breakdown during high-intensity exercise.

- Sources: Supplements.

5. HMB (Beta-Hydroxy Beta-Methylbutyrate)
   - Function: Supports muscle protein synthesis and reduces muscle breakdown.
   - Sources: Supplements.
6. Taurine
   - Function: Supports muscle contraction and reduces muscle damage during high-intensity exercise.
   - Sources: Meat, fish, dairy products, supplements.
7. Whey Protein
   - Function: Provides essential amino acids that support muscle repair and growth.
   - Sources: Dairy products, supplements.
8. Omega-3 Fatty Acids
   - Function: Reduce inflammation and support muscle recovery and endurance.
   - Sources: Fish oil, flaxseed oil, chia seeds, walnuts, supplements.

Sarcomeres: Structure and Function

Definition and Overview

Sarcomeres are the basic functional units of striated muscle fibers (both skeletal and cardiac muscles). They are the regions of the myofibrils that contract and generate force. Each sarcomere is delineated by Z-lines and composed of interlocking thick and thin filaments.

Structure of Sarcomeres

- Z-Line (Z-Disc):
    - Defines the boundaries of each sarcomere.
    - Anchors the thin (actin) filaments and connects adjacent sarcomeres.
- A-Band:

- The dark region of the sarcomere that contains the entire length of the thick (myosin) filaments.
    - Includes overlapping thick and thin filaments, contributing to muscle contraction.
- I-Band:
    - The light region on either side of the Z-line, containing only thin filaments.
    - Shortens during muscle contraction.
- H-Zone:
    - The central part of the A-Band where there are only thick filaments, without overlapping thin filaments.
    - Shortens during muscle contraction.
- M-Line:
    - Located in the center of the H-Zone.
    - Consists of proteins that hold the thick filaments together.
- Thick Filaments (Myosin):
    - Composed of myosin molecules with protruding heads that form cross-bridges with actin filaments during contraction.

- Thin Filaments (Actin):
    - Composed of actin molecules arranged in a double helix.
    - Also contain regulatory proteins tropomyosin and troponin.

Function of Sarcomeres

- Muscle Contraction:
    - Sliding Filament Theory: Explains muscle contraction. Myosin heads attach to actin filaments, pulling them toward the center of the sarcomere, causing the sarcomere to shorten.
    - ATP Role: ATP binds to myosin heads, providing the energy for the cross-bridge cycle, enabling the myosin heads to attach, pivot, detach, and reset.
- Force Generation:
    - The coordinated shortening of multiple sarcomeres along a myofibril generates significant force, resulting in muscle contraction.

Regulation of Contraction

- Calcium Ions (Ca^{2+}):
    - Released from the sarcoplasmic reticulum in response to a nerve impulse.
    - Bind to troponin, causing a conformational change that moves tropomyosin away from actin's binding sites, allowing myosin to attach.
- Troponin and Tropomyosin:
    - Tropomyosin: Blocks myosin-binding sites on actin when the muscle is relaxed.
    - Troponin: A complex of three proteins that binds to calcium ions, moving tropomyosin and exposing binding sites on actin for myosin.

Disorders Related to Sarcomeres

- Muscular Dystrophy:
    - Genetic disorders that weaken muscle fibers due to defects in

proteins that support sarcomere
structure and function.
- Cardiomyopathies:
    - Diseases of the heart muscle that
      can involve abnormalities in
      sarcomere proteins, affecting
      heart contraction and function.

Sarcomere Adaptation and Plasticity

- Hypertrophy:
    - Increase in the size of muscle
      fibers due to an increase in the
      number of myofibrils, including
      sarcomeres, within each muscle
      cell.
    - Common in response to
      resistance training and strength
      training.
- Hyperplasia:
    - Increase in the number of muscle
      fibers, contributing to muscle
      growth, although this is less
      common than hypertrophy.

Sarcomeres are the fundamental contractile units of striated muscle fibers, composed of interlocking thick and thin filaments that slide past each other to produce muscle contraction. They are structured with distinct regions (Z-line, A-Band, I-Band, H-Zone, and M-Line) and regulated by calcium ions and regulatory proteins (troponin and tropomyosin). The proper function of sarcomeres is crucial for muscle force generation and movement, and their health can be affected by various genetic and acquired disorders. Understanding sarcomeres is essential for comprehending how muscles contract, adapt, and respond to different stimuli.

Herbs, Vitamins, Minerals, and Supplements for Supporting Sarcomeres

Maintaining the health and function of sarcomeres is essential for muscle contraction, repair, and overall performance. Here are some key nutrients, herbs, and supplements that contribute to the maintenance and enhancement of sarcomeres:

Vitamins

1. Vitamin D
    - Function: Enhances calcium absorption, crucial for muscle contraction and proper sarcomere function.
    - Sources: Sunlight, fortified dairy products, fatty fish, supplements.
2. Vitamin E
    - Function: Acts as an antioxidant, protecting muscle cells from oxidative stress and damage.
    - Sources: Nuts, seeds, spinach, vegetable oils, supplements.
3. Vitamin C

- Function: Essential for collagen synthesis, important for muscle repair and connective tissue health.
- Sources: Citrus fruits, strawberries, bell peppers, broccoli, kiwi, supplements.

4. Vitamin B6 (Pyridoxine)
   - Function: Important for protein metabolism and muscle growth.
   - Sources: Poultry, fish, potatoes, chickpeas, bananas, supplements.

5. Vitamin B12 (Cobalamin)
   - Function: Supports red blood cell formation and oxygen transport, crucial for muscle performance.
   - Sources: Meat, fish, dairy products, eggs, fortified cereals, supplements.

Minerals

1. Magnesium
   - Function: Essential for muscle relaxation and energy production, helps prevent cramps and muscle fatigue.

- Sources: Leafy green vegetables, nuts, seeds, whole grains, legumes, supplements.

2. Calcium
   - Function: Vital for muscle contraction and signaling within muscle cells.
   - Sources: Dairy products, fortified plant-based milks, leafy green vegetables, supplements.

3. Zinc
   - Function: Supports protein synthesis and muscle repair.
   - Sources: Meat, shellfish, legumes, seeds, nuts, supplements.

4. Iron
   - Function: Important for oxygen transport in the blood, essential for muscle performance and endurance.
   - Sources: Red meat, poultry, fish, lentils, beans, spinach, supplements.

Herbs

1. Ashwagandha (Withania somnifera)

- Function: Adaptogen that helps increase strength, reduce fatigue, and improve muscle recovery.
- Uses: Capsules, extracts, teas.

2. Ginseng (Panax ginseng)
   - Function: Enhances physical performance and reduces fatigue, supporting muscle strength and endurance.
   - Uses: Capsules, extracts, teas.

3. Turmeric (Curcuma longa)
   - Function: Contains curcumin, which has anti-inflammatory properties that support muscle recovery.
   - Uses: Fresh root, powder, capsules, extracts.

4. Rhodiola (Rhodiola rosea)
   - Function: Improves endurance and reduces fatigue by enhancing oxygen utilization.
   - Uses: Capsules, extracts, teas.

5. Eleuthero (Eleutherococcus senticosus)
   - Function: Increases stamina and reduces fatigue, supporting high-intensity muscle performance.
   - Uses: Capsules, extracts, teas.

Supplements

1. Creatine Monohydrate
   - Function: Enhances ATP production, improves muscle strength, power, and performance during high-intensity activities.
   - Sources: Supplements.
2. Beta-Alanine
   - Function: Helps buffer acid in muscles, improving endurance and reducing fatigue during high-intensity activities.
   - Sources: Supplements.
3. L-Arginine
   - Function: Precursor to nitric oxide, which improves blood flow to muscles, enhancing oxygen delivery and muscle performance.
   - Sources: Supplements.
4. Branched-Chain Amino Acids (BCAAs)
   - Function: Support muscle protein synthesis and reduce muscle breakdown during high-intensity exercise.
   - Sources: Supplements.
5. HMB (Beta-Hydroxy Beta-Methylbutyrate)

- Function: Supports muscle
  protein synthesis and reduces
  muscle breakdown.
- Sources: Supplements.

6. Taurine
  - Function: Supports muscle
    contraction and reduces muscle
    damage during high-intensity
    exercise.
  - Sources: Meat, fish, dairy
    products, supplements.

7. Whey Protein
  - Function: Provides essential
    amino acids that support muscle
    repair and growth.
  - Sources: Dairy products,
    supplements.

8. Omega-3 Fatty Acids
  - Function: Reduce inflammation
    and support muscle recovery and
    endurance.
  - Sources: Fish oil, flaxseed oil,
    chia seeds, walnuts, supplements

Sarcolemma: Structure and Function

Definition and Overview

The sarcolemma is the specialized cell membrane that surrounds muscle fibers (muscle cells). It plays a crucial role in muscle contraction by transmitting electrical impulses and maintaining the structural integrity of the muscle cell.

Structure of the Sarcolemma

- Lipid Bilayer:
    - Composed of a double layer of phospholipids, similar to other cell membranes.
    - Provides a semi-permeable barrier that regulates the entry and exit of substances.
- Integral and Peripheral Proteins:
    - Integral Proteins: Embedded within the lipid bilayer; include channels, transporters, and receptors.

- Peripheral Proteins: Attached to the inner or outer surface of the membrane; involved in signaling and structural support.
- Glycoproteins and Glycolipids:
  - Located on the extracellular surface.
  - Involved in cell recognition, communication, and interaction with the extracellular matrix.
- Dystrophin-Glycoprotein Complex:
  - Links the cytoskeleton of the muscle cell to the extracellular matrix.
  - Provides structural stability and helps transmit force generated by muscle contractions.

Functions of the Sarcolemma

- Electrical Excitability:
  - Action Potential Transmission: The sarcolemma propagates action potentials, which are electrical impulses that trigger muscle contractions.
  - Voltage-Gated Ion Channels: Control the flow of ions such as

sodium (Na+), potassium (K+),
and calcium (Ca2+), essential for
generating and propagating
action potentials.
- Structural Integrity and Support:
    - Maintains the shape and integrity
      of the muscle fiber.
    - Connects the muscle fiber to the
      extracellular matrix and other
      cells, ensuring coordinated
      contractions.
- Signal Transduction:
    - Contains receptors and signaling
      molecules that respond to
      hormones, neurotransmitters,
      and other stimuli.
    - Initiates intracellular signaling
      pathways that regulate muscle
      growth, repair, and adaptation.
- Transport of Nutrients and Waste:
    - Regulates the transport of
      nutrients, ions, and waste
      products into and out of the
      muscle cell.
    - Involves various transporters,
      pumps, and channels embedded
      in the membrane.

Disorders Related to the Sarcolemma

- Duchenne Muscular Dystrophy (DMD):
    - A genetic disorder caused by mutations in the dystrophin gene.
    - Leads to the absence of dystrophin, compromising the structural integrity of the sarcolemma and resulting in muscle weakness and degeneration.
- Becker Muscular Dystrophy (BMD):
    - Similar to DMD but caused by mutations that allow for some functional dystrophin.
    - Results in milder symptoms compared to DMD.

Sarcolemma Adaptation and Plasticity

- Exercise-Induced Adaptations:
    - Regular exercise, especially resistance training, can enhance the structural and functional properties of the sarcolemma.
    - Increases the expression of proteins involved in signal

transduction, nutrient transport,
and structural support.
- Injury and Repair:
    - The sarcolemma can repair minor
      damage through membrane
      resealing mechanisms.
    - Severe damage triggers a repair
      response involving satellite cells
      (muscle stem cells) and various
      growth factors.

The sarcolemma is the specialized cell membrane of muscle fibers, essential for transmitting electrical impulses, maintaining structural integrity, and regulating the exchange of substances. Its components, including the lipid bilayer, proteins, glycoproteins, and the dystrophin-glycoprotein complex, play vital roles in muscle function. The sarcolemma's ability to adapt to exercise and repair damage is crucial for muscle health, and its dysfunction can lead to severe muscle disorders like Duchenne and Becker muscular dystrophies. Understanding the sarcolemma is key to comprehending muscle physiology, pathology, and the effects of various interventions on muscle health.

Herbs, Vitamins, Minerals, and Supplements for Supporting the Sarcolemma

The sarcolemma's health is crucial for muscle contraction, signaling, and overall muscle function. Here are some key nutrients, herbs, and supplements that contribute to the maintenance and enhancement of the sarcolemma:

Vitamins

1. Vitamin D
   - Function: Enhances calcium absorption, crucial for muscle function and overall cellular health.
   - Sources: Sunlight, fortified dairy products, fatty fish, supplements.
2. Vitamin E
   - Function: Acts as an antioxidant, protecting the sarcolemma from oxidative stress and damage.
   - Sources: Nuts, seeds, spinach, vegetable oils, supplements.
3. Vitamin C

- Function: Essential for collagen synthesis, important for the structural integrity of the sarcolemma and connective tissue.
  - Sources: Citrus fruits, strawberries, bell peppers, broccoli, kiwi, supplements.
4. Vitamin B6 (Pyridoxine)
  - Function: Important for protein metabolism and muscle health.
  - Sources: Poultry, fish, potatoes, chickpeas, bananas, supplements.
5. Vitamin B12 (Cobalamin)
  - Function: Supports red blood cell formation and oxygen transport, crucial for muscle performance.
  - Sources: Meat, fish, dairy products, eggs, fortified cereals, supplements.

Minerals

1. Magnesium
  - Function: Essential for muscle relaxation, energy production, and maintaining cell membrane integrity.

- Sources: Leafy green vegetables, nuts, seeds, whole grains, legumes, supplements.

2. Calcium
   - Function: Vital for muscle contraction and signaling within muscle cells.
   - Sources: Dairy products, fortified plant-based milks, leafy green vegetables, supplements.

3. Zinc
   - Function: Supports protein synthesis, cell membrane repair, and muscle health.
   - Sources: Meat, shellfish, legumes, seeds, nuts, supplements.

4. Iron
   - Function: Important for oxygen transport in the blood, essential for muscle performance and endurance.
   - Sources: Red meat, poultry, fish, lentils, beans, spinach, supplements.

Herbs

1. Ashwagandha (Withania somnifera)

- Function: Adaptogen that helps
  increase strength, reduce fatigue,
  and improve muscle recovery.
- Uses: Capsules, extracts, teas.

2. Ginseng (Panax ginseng)
   - Function: Enhances physical
     performance and reduces fatigue,
     supporting muscle strength and
     endurance.
   - Uses: Capsules, extracts, teas.

3. Turmeric (Curcuma longa)
   - Function: Contains curcumin,
     which has anti-inflammatory
     properties that support muscle
     recovery.
   - Uses: Fresh root, powder,
     capsules, extracts.

4. Rhodiola (Rhodiola rosea)
   - Function: Improves endurance
     and reduces fatigue by enhancing
     oxygen utilization.
   - Uses: Capsules, extracts, teas.

5. Eleuthero (Eleutherococcus senticosus)
   - Function: Increases stamina and
     reduces fatigue, supporting
     high-intensity muscle
     performance.
   - Uses: Capsules, extracts, teas.

Supplements

1. Creatine Monohydrate
   - Function: Enhances ATP production, improves muscle strength, power, and performance during high-intensity activities.
   - Sources: Supplements.
2. Beta-Alanine
   - Function: Helps buffer acid in muscles, improving endurance and reducing fatigue during high-intensity activities.
   - Sources: Supplements.
3. L-Arginine
   - Function: Precursor to nitric oxide, which improves blood flow to muscles, enhancing oxygen delivery and muscle performance.
   - Sources: Supplements.
4. Branched-Chain Amino Acids (BCAAs)
   - Function: Support muscle protein synthesis and reduce muscle breakdown during high-intensity exercise.
   - Sources: Supplements.
5. HMB (Beta-Hydroxy Beta-Methylbutyrate)

- Function: Supports muscle
     protein synthesis and reduces
     muscle breakdown.
   - Sources: Supplements.
6. Taurine
   - Function: Supports muscle
     contraction and reduces muscle
     damage during high-intensity
     exercise.
   - Sources: Meat, fish, dairy
     products, supplements.
7. Whey Protein
   - Function: Provides essential
     amino acids that support muscle
     repair and growth.
   - Sources: Dairy products,
     supplements.
8. Omega-3 Fatty Acids
   - Function: Reduce inflammation
     and support muscle recovery and
     endurance.
   - Sources: Fish oil, flaxseed oil,
     chia seeds, walnuts, supplements.

Sarcoplasm: Structure and Function

Definition and Overview

The sarcoplasm is the cytoplasm of a muscle fiber (muscle cell). It is a gel-like substance that fills the interior of the muscle cell, surrounding the myofibrils (contractile elements) and housing various organelles and other structures necessary for muscle function.

Structure of the Sarcoplasm

- Cytoplasmic Components:
    - Contains a mixture of water, proteins, fats, glycogen, and various ions.
    - Suspends organelles such as mitochondria, the sarcoplasmic reticulum, and ribosomes.
- Organelles:
    - Mitochondria: The powerhouse of the cell, providing ATP through oxidative phosphorylation.
    - Sarcoplasmic Reticulum (SR): A specialized type of smooth

endoplasmic reticulum that
stores and releases calcium ions
(Ca^{2+}), crucial for muscle
contraction.
  - Ribosomes: Sites of protein
    synthesis.
- Other Structures:
  - Myoglobin: An oxygen-binding
    protein that stores and transports
    oxygen within muscle cells.
  - Glycogen Granules: Serve as a
    storage form of glucose,
    providing energy during muscle
    activity.
  - Enzymes: Various enzymes
    involved in metabolic processes,
    including glycolysis and the
    Krebs cycle.

Functions of the Sarcoplasm

- Energy Production:
  - ATP Synthesis: Mitochondria
    within the sarcoplasm produce
    ATP, the primary energy source
    for muscle contraction.

- Glycolysis: The breakdown of
    glucose to pyruvate, producing
    ATP anaerobically.
  - Glycogenolysis: The breakdown
    of glycogen to glucose, supplying
    energy during intense muscle
    activity.
- Calcium Storage and Release:
  - The sarcoplasmic reticulum (SR)
    within the sarcoplasm stores
    calcium ions and releases them in
    response to an action potential,
    initiating muscle contraction.
- Oxygen Storage and Transport:
  - Myoglobin: Binds oxygen and
    facilitates its diffusion to the
    mitochondria, especially during
    periods of intense muscle activity.
- Metabolic Activities:
  - Hosts various metabolic
    pathways and enzymes necessary
    for energy production and muscle
    function.

Disorders Related to the Sarcoplasm

- Metabolic Myopathies:

- Disorders that affect the
    metabolic processes within
    muscle cells, often due to enzyme
    deficiencies, leading to muscle
    weakness and fatigue.
  - Mitochondrial Myopathies:
    - Genetic disorders affecting the
      function of mitochondria,
      resulting in impaired energy
      production and muscle weakness.

Adaptation and Plasticity

- Exercise-Induced Changes:
  - Endurance Training: Increases
    the number and efficiency of
    mitochondria, enhancing the
    muscle's oxidative capacity.
  - Resistance Training: Promotes
    glycogen storage and increases
    the activity of glycolytic enzymes,
    improving anaerobic energy
    production.
- Nutritional Influences:
  - Adequate intake of nutrients such
    as carbohydrates, fats, and
    proteins supports the energy

demands of the muscle and the synthesis of ATP.

The sarcoplasm is the cytoplasm of muscle fibers, encompassing various organelles and structures essential for muscle function. It plays a vital role in energy production, calcium storage and release, oxygen storage and transport, and various metabolic activities. Proper functioning of the sarcoplasm is crucial for muscle contraction, endurance, and overall performance. Understanding the sarcoplasm's components and functions is key to comprehending how muscles produce energy, respond to stimuli, and adapt to different types of physical activity.

Herbs, Vitamins, Minerals, and Supplements for Supporting Sarcoplasm

The sarcoplasm is essential for muscle energy production, calcium handling, and overall muscle function. To maintain and enhance the health of the sarcoplasm, specific nutrients, herbs, and supplements can be beneficial.

Vitamins

1. Vitamin D
    - Function: Enhances calcium absorption, which is vital for muscle contraction and overall cellular function.
    - Sources: Sunlight, fortified dairy products, fatty fish, supplements.
2. Vitamin E
    - Function: Acts as an antioxidant, protecting muscle cells from oxidative stress and damage.
    - Sources: Nuts, seeds, spinach, vegetable oils, supplements.
3. Vitamin C
    - Function: Essential for collagen synthesis, which supports muscle tissue integrity and repair.
    - Sources: Citrus fruits, strawberries, bell peppers, broccoli, kiwi, supplements.
4. Vitamin B6 (Pyridoxine)
    - Function: Important for protein metabolism and muscle function.

- Sources: Poultry, fish, potatoes, chickpeas, bananas, supplements.

5. Vitamin B12 (Cobalamin)
   - Function: Supports red blood cell formation and oxygen transport, crucial for muscle performance.
   - Sources: Meat, fish, dairy products, eggs, fortified cereals, supplements.

Minerals

1. Magnesium
   - Function: Essential for muscle relaxation, energy production, and maintaining cell membrane integrity.
   - Sources: Leafy green vegetables, nuts, seeds, whole grains, legumes, supplements.
2. Calcium
   - Function: Vital for muscle contraction and signaling within muscle cells.
   - Sources: Dairy products, fortified plant-based milks, leafy green vegetables, supplements.
3. Zinc

- Function: Supports protein
  synthesis, cell membrane repair,
  and muscle health.
- Sources: Meat, shellfish, legumes,
  seeds, nuts, supplements.

4. Iron
   - Function: Important for oxygen
     transport in the blood, essential
     for muscle performance and
     endurance.
   - Sources: Red meat, poultry, fish,
     lentils, beans, spinach,
     supplements.

Herbs

1. Ashwagandha (Withania somnifera)
   - Function: Adaptogen that helps
     increase strength, reduce fatigue,
     and improve muscle recovery.
   - Uses: Capsules, extracts, teas.
2. Ginseng (Panax ginseng)
   - Function: Enhances physical
     performance and reduces fatigue,
     supporting muscle strength and
     endurance.
   - Uses: Capsules, extracts, teas.
3. Turmeric (Curcuma longa)

- Function: Contains curcumin,
      which has anti-inflammatory
      properties that support muscle
      recovery.
    - Uses: Fresh root, powder,
      capsules, extracts.
4. Rhodiola (Rhodiola rosea)
    - Function: Improves endurance
      and reduces fatigue by enhancing
      oxygen utilization.
    - Uses: Capsules, extracts, teas.
5. Eleuthero (Eleutherococcus senticosus)
    - Function: Increases stamina and
      reduces fatigue, supporting
      high-intensity muscle
      performance.
    - Uses: Capsules, extracts, teas.

Supplements

1. Creatine Monohydrate
    - Function: Enhances ATP
      production, improves muscle
      strength, power, and
      performance during
      high-intensity activities.
    - Sources: Supplements.
2. Beta-Alanine

- Function: Helps buffer acid in muscles, improving endurance and reducing fatigue during high-intensity activities.
  - Sources: Supplements.
3. L-Arginine
   - Function: Precursor to nitric oxide, which improves blood flow to muscles, enhancing oxygen delivery and muscle performance.
   - Sources: Supplements.
4. Branched-Chain Amino Acids (BCAAs)
   - Function: Support muscle protein synthesis and reduce muscle breakdown during high-intensity exercise.
   - Sources: Supplements.
5. HMB (Beta-Hydroxy Beta-Methylbutyrate)
   - Function: Supports muscle protein synthesis and reduces muscle breakdown.
   - Sources: Supplements.
6. Taurine
   - Function: Supports muscle contraction and reduces muscle damage during high-intensity exercise.

- Sources: Meat, fish, dairy products, supplements.

7. Whey Protein
    - Function: Provides essential amino acids that support muscle repair and growth.
    - Sources: Dairy products, supplements.
8. Omega-3 Fatty Acids
    - Function: Reduce inflammation and support muscle recovery and endurance.
    - Sources: Fish oil, flaxseed oil, chia seeds, walnuts, supplements.

Lifestyle Practices

1. Regular Exercise
    - Importance: Stimulates the growth and strength of muscle fibers and enhances sarcoplasmic health.
    - Types: Weight training, resistance training, high-intensity interval training (HIIT).
2. Balanced Diet
    - Focus: A diet rich in lean proteins, healthy fats, complex

carbohydrates, fruits, and
vegetables supports overall
muscle health.
- Avoid: Excessive intake of
processed foods, high-sodium
foods, and sugar.
3. Adequate Hydration
- Importance: Maintains muscle
function and prevents cramps.
- Advice: Drink plenty of water
throughout the day.
4. Adequate Sleep
- Importance: Essential for muscle
recovery and repair.
- Advice: Aim for 7-9 hours of
quality sleep per night.

Sarcoplasmic Reticulum: Structure and Function

The sarcoplasmic reticulum (SR) is a specialized type of endoplasmic reticulum found in muscle cells, primarily skeletal and cardiac muscle fibers. It plays a crucial role in regulating calcium ion (Ca^{2+}) levels within the muscle cell, which is essential for muscle contraction and relaxation.

Structure of the Sarcoplasmic Reticulum

- Network of Tubules: The SR consists of a complex network of membrane-bound tubules that extend throughout the muscle fiber.
- Terminal Cisternae: Enlarged regions of the SR located adjacent to the T-tubules (transverse tubules), forming structures known as triads in skeletal muscle cells. These terminal cisternae are sites of calcium storage and release.
- Membrane Proteins: The SR membrane contains various proteins involved in calcium regulation, including calcium pumps (SERCA pumps), calcium channels, and calcium-binding proteins such as calsequestrin.

Function of the Sarcoplasmic Reticulum

1. Calcium Storage: The primary function of the SR is to store calcium ions (Ca^{2+}) in its terminal cisternae. Calcium is actively pumped into the SR lumen by sarco/endoplasmic reticulum calcium ATPase (SERCA) pumps, creating a high concentration gradient.

2. Calcium Release: When a muscle fiber is stimulated to contract, an action potential travels along the sarcolemma (muscle cell membrane) and into the T-tubules. This triggers the opening of voltage-gated calcium channels in the T-tubule membrane, leading to a rapid influx of calcium ions. The change in membrane potential then activates calcium release channels called ryanodine receptors (RYR) in the adjacent terminal cisternae of the SR. These channels release stored calcium ions into the sarcoplasm (cytoplasm), initiating muscle contraction.

3. Calcium Reuptake: After muscle contraction, calcium ions need to be rapidly removed from the cytoplasm to allow the muscle to relax. SERCA pumps actively transport calcium ions back into the SR, lowering cytoplasmic calcium

levels and allowing the muscle to return to its resting state.

4. Regulation of Muscle Contraction: By controlling the availability of calcium ions in the cytoplasm, the sarcoplasmic reticulum regulates the contraction and relaxation of muscle fibers. Proper regulation ensures coordinated muscle activity and prevents sustained contraction (tetany) or prolonged relaxation.

Disorders Related to the Sarcoplasmic Reticulum

- Malignant Hyperthermia: A rare but potentially life-threatening condition triggered by certain drugs that cause uncontrolled release of calcium from the SR, leading to muscle rigidity, high fever, and metabolic disturbances.
- Central Core Disease: A congenital muscle disorder associated with mutations in genes encoding proteins involved in SR function, resulting in muscle weakness and structural abnormalities.

Adaptation and Plasticity

- Exercise-induced Changes: Regular physical activity can lead to adaptations in the sarcoplasmic reticulum, including increased calcium storage capacity and enhanced calcium handling, which contribute to improved muscle performance and endurance.
- Nutritional Influences: Adequate intake of nutrients such as calcium, magnesium, and vitamin D supports the proper function of the sarcoplasmic reticulum and muscle contraction.

Understanding the structure and function of the sarcoplasmic reticulum is essential for comprehending muscle physiology, contraction mechanisms, and the impact of various factors on muscle performance and health.

Herbs, Vitamins, Minerals, and Supplements for Supporting Sarcoplasmic Reticulum Function

Maintaining the health and function of the sarcoplasmic reticulum (SR) is crucial for proper muscle contraction and relaxation. Here are some nutrients, herbs, and supplements that support SR function:

Vitamins

1. Vitamin D
    - Function: Supports calcium absorption and utilization, essential for proper SR function.
    - Sources: Sunlight exposure, fortified dairy products, fatty fish, supplements.
2. Vitamin C
    - Function: Acts as an antioxidant, protecting SR membranes from oxidative damage.
    - Sources: Citrus fruits, strawberries, bell peppers, broccoli, supplements.

Minerals

1. Calcium
    - Function: Essential for SR calcium storage and release, crucial for muscle contraction.

- Sources: Dairy products, leafy greens, fortified foods, supplements.

2. Magnesium
   - Function: Supports SR function by regulating calcium flux and muscle relaxation.
   - Sources: Nuts, seeds, whole grains, leafy greens, supplements.

Supplements

1. Creatine
   - Function: Enhances ATP production, supporting SR calcium reuptake and muscle contraction.
   - Sources: Creatine monohydrate supplements.
2. Coenzyme Q10 (CoQ10)
   - Function: Supports mitochondrial function and energy production, important for SR activity.
   - Sources: Fish, meat, nuts, seeds, supplements.
3. L-Carnitine

- Function: Facilitates the transport of fatty acids into mitochondria for energy production, supporting SR function indirectly.
- Sources: Red meat, fish, poultry, supplements.

Herbs

1. Ginseng (Panax ginseng)
   - Function: Adaptogen with potential benefits for muscle function and energy metabolism, supporting SR health indirectly.
   - Forms: Capsules, extracts, teas.
2. Rhodiola (Rhodiola rosea)
   - Function: Enhances energy production and physical performance, potentially supporting SR function.
   - Forms: Capsules, extracts, teas.

Endomysium: Structure and Function

The endomysium is a delicate layer of connective tissue that surrounds individual muscle fibers (muscle cells) within a muscle. It plays several important roles in supporting muscle function and integrity.

Structure of the Endomysium

- Composition: The endomysium is primarily composed of collagen fibers, a type of structural protein that provides strength and support to tissues.
- Delicacy: Compared to the perimysium (connective tissue surrounding bundles of muscle fibers) and epimysium (connective tissue surrounding entire muscles), the endomysium is the thinnest and most delicate layer of connective tissue within muscle tissue.
- Blood Supply and Nerve Fibers: While sparse, the endomysium contains capillaries (tiny blood vessels) and nerve endings that supply nutrients and signals to individual muscle fibers.

Function of the Endomysium

1. Support and Protection: The endomysium provides physical support and protection to individual muscle fibers, helping to maintain their structural integrity during contraction and movement.
2. Facilitation of Contraction: By surrounding each muscle fiber, the endomysium allows for independent movement and contraction of individual fibers, contributing to the overall coordinated movement of the muscle.
3. Provision of Nutrients and Oxygen: Capillaries within the endomysium supply oxygen and nutrients to the muscle fibers, essential for energy production and muscle function.
4. Waste Removal: Capillaries also facilitate the removal of metabolic waste products, such as carbon dioxide and lactic acid, from the muscle fibers, promoting optimal muscle function and recovery.
5. Transmission of Signals: Nerve endings within the endomysium transmit signals from the nervous system to the muscle fibers, coordinating muscle contractions and movements.

Disorders Related to the Endomysium

- Muscle Atrophy: Conditions that lead to muscle wasting and atrophy can also affect the endomysium, compromising its ability to support and protect muscle fibers.
- Muscle Strains and Tears: Injuries to muscles, such as strains and tears, can damage the endomysium, leading to inflammation and impaired muscle function.

Adaptation and Plasticity

- Exercise-Induced Changes: Regular exercise, particularly resistance training, can stimulate adaptations within the endomysium, promoting its strength and resilience.
- Nutritional Support: Adequate intake of nutrients such as protein, collagen, and vitamins supports the synthesis and maintenance of connective tissues like the endomysium.

Understanding the structure and function of the endomysium is essential for comprehending

Herbs, Vitamins, Minerals, and Supplements for Supporting Endomysium Health

Maintaining the health and integrity of the endomysium is crucial for optimal muscle function and performance. Here are some nutrients, herbs, and supplements that can support endomysium health:

Vitamins

1. Vitamin C
   - Function: Promotes collagen synthesis, essential for the formation and repair of connective tissues like the endomysium.
   - Sources: Citrus fruits, bell peppers, strawberries, broccoli, supplements.
2. Vitamin E
   - Function: Acts as an antioxidant, protecting connective tissues

from oxidative damage and
supporting their health.
- Sources: Nuts, seeds, spinach,
avocado, vegetable oils,
supplements.

Minerals

1. Calcium
    - Function: Supports the structural
      integrity of connective tissues,
      including the endomysium.
    - Sources: Dairy products, leafy
      greens, fortified foods,
      supplements.
2. Magnesium
    - Function: Essential for collagen
      formation and muscle function,
      supporting endomysium health
      indirectly.
    - Sources: Nuts, seeds, whole
      grains, leafy greens, supplements.

Supplements

1. Collagen
   - Function: Provides the building blocks for connective tissues like the endomysium, promoting their strength and resilience.
   - Sources: Collagen supplements derived from animal sources (e.g., bovine collagen, marine collagen).
2. Omega-3 Fatty Acids
   - Function: Have anti-inflammatory properties, supporting the health of connective tissues and reducing inflammation in the endomysium.
   - Sources: Fatty fish (salmon, mackerel, sardines), flaxseeds, chia seeds, fish oil supplements.

Herbs

1. Turmeric (Curcuma longa)
   - Function: Contains curcumin, which has anti-inflammatory properties that can support endomysium health.

- Forms: Fresh turmeric root,
  ground turmeric powder,
  turmeric supplements.
2. Ginger (Zingiber officinale)
   - Function: Has anti-inflammatory
     and antioxidant effects,
     potentially benefiting connective
     tissues like the endomysium.
   - Forms: Fresh ginger root, ginger
     tea, ginger supplements.

Lifestyle Practices

1. Adequate Hydration
   - Importance: Proper hydration
     supports the health and elasticity
     of connective tissues, including
     the endomysium.
   - Advice: Drink plenty of water
     throughout the day, especially
     before and after exercise.
2. Balanced Diet
   - Focus: Consume a diet rich in
     fruits, vegetables, lean proteins,
     and whole grains to provide
     essential nutrients for connective
     tissue health.

- Include: Foods rich in vitamin C, vitamin E, calcium, magnesium, and omega-3 fatty acids.
3. Regular Exercise
    - Importance: Exercise stimulates collagen synthesis and promotes overall tissue health, including the endomysium.
    - Types: Resistance training, flexibility exercises, cardiovascular exercise.
4. Stress Management
    - Importance: Chronic stress can contribute to inflammation and oxidative damage, negatively impacting connective tissue health.
    - Practices: Practice stress-reducing techniques such as meditation, deep breathing, yoga, and adequate rest.

Perimysium: Structure and Function

The perimysium is a layer of connective tissue that surrounds bundles of muscle fibers within skeletal muscles. It plays several important roles in supporting muscle function and facilitating coordinated movement.

Structure of the Perimysium

- Composition: The perimysium is composed of collagen fibers, elastic fibers, and fibroblasts (connective tissue cells) arranged in a dense, irregular pattern.
- Surrounding Muscle Bundles: Muscle fibers are organized into bundles called fascicles, each surrounded by a layer of perimysium. The perimysium divides the muscle into distinct compartments, providing structural support and organization.
- Blood Supply and Nerve Supply: The perimysium contains blood vessels and nerve fibers that supply nutrients and signals to the muscle fibers within the fascicles.

Function of the Perimysium

1. Mechanical Support: The perimysium provides structural support and protection to the bundles of muscle fibers, helping to maintain their integrity during contraction and movement.
2. Transmission of Force: By transmitting forces generated by muscle contractions, the perimysium helps to distribute tension evenly throughout the muscle, ensuring efficient movement and minimizing the risk of injury.
3. Compartmentalization: By dividing the muscle into compartments (fascicles), the perimysium allows for the independent contraction of muscle fibers within each fascicle, contributing to the overall coordinated movement of the muscle.
4. Blood and Nerve Supply: Blood vessels within the perimysium deliver oxygen and nutrients to the muscle fibers, while nerve fibers transmit signals from the nervous system to control muscle contraction and relaxation.

Disorders Related to the Perimysium

- Muscle Strains: Injuries such as muscle strains or tears can damage the perimysium, leading to inflammation and impaired muscle function.
- Compartment Syndrome: Increased pressure within the compartments formed by the perimysium can result in compartment syndrome, a painful condition that affects blood flow and nerve function in the affected area.

Adaptation and Plasticity

- Exercise-Induced Changes: Regular exercise, particularly resistance training, can stimulate adaptations within the perimysium, promoting its strength and resilience.
- Nutritional Support: Adequate intake of nutrients such as protein, collagen, and vitamins supports the synthesis and maintenance of connective tissues like the perimysium.

Herbs, Vitamins, Minerals, and Supplements for Supporting Perimysium Health

Maintaining the health and integrity of the perimysium is crucial for optimal muscle function and performance. Here are some nutrients, herbs, and supplements that can support perimysium health:

Vitamins

1. Vitamin C
    - Function: Promotes collagen synthesis, essential for the formation and repair of connective tissues like the perimysium.
    - Sources: Citrus fruits, bell peppers, strawberries, broccoli, supplements.
2. Vitamin E
    - Function: Acts as an antioxidant, protecting connective tissues from oxidative damage and supporting their health.

- Sources: Nuts, seeds, spinach, avocado, vegetable oils, supplements.

Minerals

1. Calcium
   - Function: Supports the structural integrity of connective tissues like the perimysium.
   - Sources: Dairy products, leafy greens, fortified foods, supplements.
2. Magnesium
   - Function: Essential for collagen formation and muscle function, indirectly supporting perimysium health.
   - Sources: Nuts, seeds, whole grains, leafy greens, supplements.

Supplements

1. Collagen
   - Function: Provides the building blocks for connective tissues like

the perimysium, promoting their strength and resilience.

- Sources: Collagen supplements derived from animal sources (e.g., bovine collagen, marine collagen).

2. Omega-3 Fatty Acids
   - Function: Have anti-inflammatory properties, supporting the health of connective tissues and reducing inflammation in the perimysium.
   - Sources: Fatty fish (salmon, mackerel, sardines), flaxseeds, chia seeds, fish oil supplements.

Herbs

1. Turmeric (Curcuma longa)
   - Function: Contains curcumin, which has anti-inflammatory properties that can support perimysium health.
   - Forms: Fresh turmeric root, ground turmeric powder, turmeric supplements.

2. Ginger (Zingiber officinale)

- **Function:** Has anti-inflammatory and antioxidant effects, potentially benefiting connective tissues like the perimysium.
- **Forms:** Fresh ginger root, ginger tea, ginger supplements.

Epimysium: Structure and Function

The epimysium is a dense layer of connective tissue that surrounds entire muscles, providing structural support and protection. It plays several crucial roles in supporting muscle function and facilitating coordinated movement.

Structure of the Epimysium

- Composition: The epimysium is composed primarily of collagen fibers, fibroblasts (connective tissue cells), and elastic fibers arranged in a dense, irregular pattern.
- Surrounding Entire Muscles: Unlike the perimysium, which surrounds bundles of muscle fibers, the epimysium surrounds entire muscles, forming a continuous sheath around the muscle tissue.
- Integration with Tendons: At the ends of muscles, the epimysium blends seamlessly with the fibrous tissue of tendons, attaching muscles to bones and

allowing for the transmission of force during muscle contraction.

Function of the Epimysium

1. Structural Support: The epimysium provides structural support and protection to entire muscles, helping to maintain their shape and integrity during contraction and movement.
2. Transmission of Force: By surrounding entire muscles, the epimysium helps to transmit forces generated by muscle contractions to the tendons and ultimately to the bones, allowing for efficient movement and locomotion.
3. Protection of Blood Vessels and Nerves: Within the epimysium, blood vessels and nerve fibers supply nutrients and signals to the muscle tissue, supporting muscle function and coordination.
4. Compartmentalization: While the epimysium surrounds entire muscles, it also helps to compartmentalize the muscle tissue, dividing it into distinct functional units and facilitating coordinated movement.

Disorders Related to the Epimysium

- Muscle Tears: Injuries such as muscle tears or strains can damage the epimysium, leading to inflammation and impaired muscle function.
- Tendinopathies: Conditions affecting tendons, such as tendinitis or tendinosis, can also involve the epimysium where tendons attach to muscles.

Adaptation and Plasticity

- Exercise-Induced Changes: Regular exercise, particularly resistance training, can stimulate adaptations within the epimysium, promoting its strength and resilience.
- Nutritional Support: Adequate intake of nutrients such as protein, collagen, and vitamins supports the synthesis and maintenance of connective tissues like the epimysium.

Herbs, Vitamins, Minerals, and Supplements for Supporting Epimysium Health

Maintaining the health and integrity of the epimysium is essential for optimal muscle function and performance. Here are some nutrients, herbs, and supplements that can support epimysium health:

Vitamins

1. Vitamin C
   - Function: Promotes collagen synthesis, essential for the formation and repair of connective tissues like the epimysium.
   - Sources: Citrus fruits, bell peppers, strawberries, broccoli, supplements.
2. Vitamin E
   - Function: Acts as an antioxidant, protecting connective tissues from oxidative damage and supporting their health.

- Sources: Nuts, seeds, spinach, avocado, vegetable oils, supplements.

Minerals

1. Calcium
   - Function: Supports the structural integrity of connective tissues like the epimysium.
   - Sources: Dairy products, leafy greens, fortified foods, supplements.
2. Magnesium
   - Function: Essential for collagen formation and muscle function, indirectly supporting epimysium health.
   - Sources: Nuts, seeds, whole grains, leafy greens, supplements.

Supplements

1. Collagen
   - Function: Provides the building blocks for connective tissues like

the epimysium, promoting their strength and resilience.
  - Sources: Collagen supplements derived from animal sources (e.g., bovine collagen, marine collagen).
2. Omega-3 Fatty Acids
  - Function: Have anti-inflammatory properties, supporting the health of connective tissues and reducing inflammation in the epimysium.
  - Sources: Fatty fish (salmon, mackerel, sardines), flaxseeds, chia seeds, fish oil supplements.

Herbs

1. Turmeric (Curcuma longa)
  - Function: Contains curcumin, which has anti-inflammatory properties that can support epimysium health.
  - Forms: Fresh turmeric root, ground turmeric powder, turmeric supplements.
2. Ginger (Zingiber officinale)

- **Function**: Has anti-inflammatory and antioxidant effects, potentially benefiting connective tissues like the epimysium.
- **Forms**: Fresh ginger root, ginger tea, ginger supplements.

Ending Thoughts

In the pages of "The Natural Path to Healing Your Muscles," you've embarked on a transformative journey towards vibrant muscle health and overall well-being. Throughout this comprehensive guide, you've delved deep into the intricate world of muscles, exploring their diverse types, essential connective tissues, and the interconnectedness of body and mind.

You've uncovered the healing power of nature, discovering a wealth of vitamins, minerals, herbs, and supplements that nourish and support your muscles from within. By embracing holistic lifestyle practices such as hydration, nutrition, movement, and mindfulness, you've cultivated a harmonious relationship with your muscles, fostering balance, resilience, and vitality.

As you've journeyed along the natural path to healing, strength, and vitality in your muscles, you've empowered yourself with knowledge, tools, and resources to take proactive control of your muscle health. With each step, you've embraced a mindset of self-awareness, self-care, and self-empowerment, knowing that you hold the keys to unlocking the innate healing potential of your body.

Now, as you reach the culmination of this transformative journey, you stand poised to embrace vibrant health and vitality in your muscles and beyond. Armed with the wisdom and insights gained from "The Natural Path to Healing Your Muscles," you're ready to navigate the natural path to holistic well-being, fostering strength, resilience, and radiant vitality in every aspect of your life.

May this guide serve as a beacon of inspiration, guidance, and support as you continue your journey towards vibrant muscle health and holistic wellness. Remember, the natural path to healing, strength, and vitality in your muscles is yours to embrace—nurture, strengthen, and thrive.

Farewell, and may your path be filled with abundant health, vitality, and joy.

Warm regards,

Luna Parnell

Legal Disclaimer

The information provided in this book, *The Natural Path to Healing Your Muscles*, is for educational and informational purposes only and is not intended as medical advice. The content of this book is based on research and personal knowledge and is meant to supplement, not replace, professional medical advice, diagnosis, or treatment.

The authors and publishers of this book are not medical professionals and do not claim to offer medical advice. Readers should consult with a qualified healthcare provider before making any decisions about their health, starting any new treatment, or discontinuing an existing treatment.

The recommendations in this book regarding herbs, vitamins, minerals, and supplements have not been evaluated by the Food and Drug Administration (FDA) and are not intended to diagnose, treat, cure, or prevent any disease. Individual results may vary, and the effectiveness of any treatment can depend on a variety of factors, including the individual's health status, age, gender, and genetic makeup.

The authors and publishers do not assume any responsibility for the misuse or misunderstanding of the information contained in this book. Any application of the advice and suggestions in this book is at the reader's discretion and sole risk.

By reading this book, you acknowledge that you understand that the information provided is not a substitute for professional medical care and that you will seek the advice of a healthcare professional for any medical concerns.

If you have any medical conditions or are taking any medications, it is crucial to consult with your healthcare provider before implementing any of the recommendations in this book.

In no event shall the authors or publishers be liable for any direct, indirect, incidental, special, or consequential damages arising out of or in connection with the use of the information contained in this book.

By using the information in this book, you agree to these terms and conditions.